INTERMITTENT FASTING

For Weight Loss And For Keto Guide

KATHERINE HAYES

Introduction

With all of the diet information online, it can be confusing to see why intermittent fasting appeals to so many people. One of the reasons why intermittent fasting is popular is because it's much easier to simply not eat periodically than to stick to a "traditional" diet.

To fast means to abstain from food and liquids (except water) for a specific duration of time. Although intermittent fasting may go against the "acceptable" ways in which we view eating in the Western world, modern science is starting to suggest that eating fewer meals and fasting more may be healthier for our body. Humans have been fasting for thousands of years. Our ancestors had to often fast for long periods since they didn't have access to plentiful food as we do now. They didn't have supermarkets and restaurants back then. If they didn't hunt for their next meal, they wouldn't be able to eat.

Fasting has also played an important role in various religions, such as Islam and Christianity. For instance, many Muslims fast for

30 days during the month of Ramadan. In addition, we fast whenever we are sleeping or sick.

If you think about it, fasting is actually quite natural. Our bodies were not made to consume food so frequently. Compared to the modern American diet, which advocates eating at least 3 large meals a day (and sometimes as many as 5-6 meals), fasting periodically may actually help to reset our body to its more natural state.

What makes intermittent fasting great is that there isn't only "one way" to do it; rather, several popular methods. A common way is the alternate-day fast, which is when a person eats normally on some days, and fasts on others. Another popular intermittent fasting method is time-restricted eating, which is when you fast at specific times during each day. We will take a closer look at the different types of intermittent fasts later on in the book.

Intermittent fasting is beneficial since it removes toxins and kick-starts your metabolism, turning your body into an effective fat-burning machine. Fasting helps to naturally reduce the body's fat by causing the metabolism to break down fat cells rather than sugar or muscle. Therefore, if you're not a fan of traditional dieting, fasting is an easy and effective way to make changes in one's physical and mental health. Other beneficial changes of fasting include alleviating minor aches and pains, increasing energy, and improving your mood.

The following chapters we will take a closer look at some of the scientific benefits of fasting and how it can be used to improve your health. Some of the topics that will be discussed include fasting's effects on your brain, human growth hormone, leptin sensitivity, insulin, and ghrelin. We will also answer commonly asked questions and examine how fasting can help those with health conditions, such as diabetes and cancer.

So, are you ready to start learning about the amazing benefits of intermittent fasting? Let's get started!

ONE

Explaining Intermittent Fasting

W hat is Intermittent Fasting about after all, and how the heck does it work? This chapter will answer these questions and more. By the end of it, you should have a solid grasp on the practice of Intermittent Fasting, and you should also have a sense of why it's trending so much these days (as well as whether or not it sounds right for you).

What it Is

Intermittent Fasting is essentially the practice of restricting mealtimes, reducing snacking, or cutting out days of eating, based on the method one chooses. One of the most popular IF methods is 5:2, which is to eat five days a week and fast the other two. Others focus on eating windows and fasting periods within each day. The easiest method to start with for IF, however, is just to stop eating snacks.

So many of us snack unconsciously or when we're getting moody without any real hunger. So many of us eat unconsciously in

1

general, and then we're confused why our bodies are holding onto the weight. Intermittent Fasting reminds the body what food is for, and it restarts that nutritional absorption potential. All you have to do is cut out the snacks, fast a few hours a day, or just drink water a few days a week.

IF is both a dietary choice and a lifestyle, but those who have the most success with IF will tell you that it became a lifestyle for them almost instantly. Sure, dieting plans and IF can match up nicely, but for some, IF requires no dietary change whatsoever. The point is to eat less and to eat less often. The brain and the body will respond in no time.

How it Works

It gives the body a break and provides a moment to recalibrate, basically. And with this recalibration, neurotransmitters are released easier in the brain, and one's senses of hungry and full are adjusted back to how they should be. Once the food is eaten after the fast, too, nutritional absorption is boosted throughout the entire body, to the benefit of all one's organs.

Additionally, Intermittent Fasting recalibrates one's hormones in relation to stress and hunger so that balanced mood, patience, and intellect can be increased despite the seeming lack of food. IF tells the brain and body to restart. It makes your system go back to basics and clean out any gunk, and a lot of that gunk tends to be stored fat or water weight. It sees the toxins in your body and refuses to let you hold onto them. Overall, IF proves that a change in routine can have great and lasting effects on one's health.

. . .

Why People Start

People most often start Intermittent Fasting because they're interested in losing that pesky and lingering weight. They're trying to lose the holiday pounds, or they're interested in slimming down for beach season. Others are trying to let go of tens, if not hundreds, of pounds through this lifestyle shift. Basically, people most often start due to weight.

On the other hand, people have been known to start IF for the sake of reversing aging, healing the heart, or healing the brain. But for now, simply know that IF can restart a lot of systems in the body, not just the digestive and endocrine systems. IF can affect the hormones that contribute to aging, the ease with which blood flows through one's veins and arteries, and the potential for the brain to heal itself with increased plasticity.

As one final point, some people start IF because they're not satisfied with the bodies they're working to sculpt at the gym. Sometimes, people aren't particularly heavy, they're just hefty, and they're working on slimming down in the right places and bulking up in others. For these people, IF can help to repurpose lingering fat to either be burned for energy or turned to muscle.

Why People Stay

People start Intermittent Fasting for a variety of reasons, but they always stay for the same reason, which is that the effects are undeniable and incredible. Regardless of why you start, you will stay because you will see changes in your body that you like, appreciate, and value. You will stay because you will have proven yourself strong in many ways and you will undoubtedly like what you've learned about yourself.

You will stay because IF will have helped you grow in ways you never imagined. Whether your goals were weight loss, anti-aging effects, sharper cognition, better memory, less disease, or otherwise, you will surely see that Intermittent Fasting can turn things around. All you need to do is devote some determination, a pinch of commitment, and a good lot of will power to the cause. Then, the sky's the limit, and your health is well within reach.

Chapter 2: The Benefits of Intermittent Fasting for Your Health

Intermittent fasting techniques, including the 16:8 method, are most commonly used to assist in weight loss by the general population. The method has been tried by thousands of people and also scientifically proven to be a helpful resource in reducing body fat and improving body composition. Weight loss is often considered the number one reason why people opt for a diet and program that utilizes intermittent fasting, in fact.

While a reduction in body fat is definitely one of the best advantages to be mentioned in terms of intermittent fasting, there are more advantages that people gain when they decide that they are going to follow this type of program – especially if they truly commit to it and can implement self-control that ensures they do not give in to cravings.

Intermittent fasting is known to assist in improving your body composition as well, as I mentioned earlier. Body composition refers to a series of features – this includes your body fat percentage and lean muscle mass primarily. A program that utilizes intermittent fasting, along with an appropriate diet plan, will bring down your body fat percentage, and push up your lean muscle mass at the same time.

It is also important to note the benefits that are associated with weight loss for people with an excessive amount of fat distributed throughout their body. Since overweight and obesity is linked to so many chronic diseases that can truly make your life dreadful, losing even small amounts of weight can drastically reduce your risk of these diseases. Additionally, if you have already been diagnosed with a disease associated with obesity, reduced body weight may improve the symptoms that you are experiencing and help you get the disease under control.

Take type 2 diabetes, for example. In one study, scientists describe that factors such as proinflammatory markers, cytokines, hormones, glycerol, and nonesterified fatty acids are all increased among those people who are obese. In turn, these factors all have factors that link them to insulin resistance. When insulin resistance develops, it can continue to progress into type 2 diabetes if the affected person does not implement appropriate preventative measures.

When you develop type 2 diabetes, you become predisposed to many additional risks and complications. In fact, type 2 diabetes can cause severe complications that may not only lead to disability but also become life-threatening. This disease can also affect all of the body's most important organs, including the heart, and can damage various tissues, such as nerves, throughout the body.

In addition to assisting in reducing body weight and bringing down the risks associated with obesity, intermittent fasting has many other benefits that are also worth mentioning.

Through intermittent fasting, cellular changes may occur in the body. This can lead to levels of human growth hormones rising by as much as 500%. This leads to a faster rate of fat burning, while also producing an increase in muscle mass.

It has also been found that intermittent fasting can help to remove waste that has built up in cells within the human body and can also assist in the repair process of cells that have been damaged. This means cells in the body become more efficient in performing their specialized functions.

One study also explains how recent findings from scientists suggest that intermittent fasting helps to improve brain health and may play a crucial role in helping medical experts better understand how diseases like Parkinson's disease and Alzheimer's disease can be prevented in the future.

Furthermore, following an intermittent fasting plan can also help to reduce levels of inflammation within the human body, as well as help to fight against oxidative stress. Both of these factors are known to contribute to numerous chronic diseases significantly and can causes certain molecules to become damaged, which can inhibit their functionality within the body.

In one study, scientists tested how intermittent fasting would work on the brain health and cardiovascular health among a group of laboratory rats. They found significant improvements in various tests used to determine the well-being of these two crucial hormones of the body. The scientists also associated these improvements among the tested laboratory rats with the reduction in oxidative stress that were observed. Additionally, the scientists also observed an improvement in the cellular stress resistance ratings in these rats. What this means is that an intermittent fasting diet can help to reduce the effect that stress has on the body, and help to fight against the existing oxidative damage, often also referred to as free radical damage, that has already occurred.

TWO

Faqs About Intermittent Fasting

I s fasting safe?

Yes, fasting is safe for most people. However, there are certain individuals who shouldn't fast. People with a serious medical condition or those who are taking medication for their blood sugar (such as insulin), must be more cautious if they are considering fasting.

If you have an eating disorder or have eating problems in the past, you should avoid intermittent fasting. The act of fasting and eating could emulate the "restricting and binging" patterns of many eating disorders, which can trigger the disorder again.

Those who should not fast include:

• Infants and children (their bodies are still growing and require more calories)

• The elderly (a restricted food diet may not be beneficial to them)

• People with diabetes

• People who are hypoglycemic

• Women who are pregnant or nursing

• Women who are trying to conceive

• Women with a history of amenorrhea

• People recovering from a major surgery or serious injury

• People who are underweight or malnourished

• People with a history of eating disorders, such as anorexia or bulimia

• People with a history of malnutrition

• Anyone with a compromised immune system

• People on certain medications, such as insulin

• People with heart complications

• People who with severe heartburn and/or GERD (gastro esophageal reflux disease)

• People who experience hypertension

• People who have issues with their blood sugar levels

• People who have low blood pressure

To ensure fasting is safe for you, consult with your doctor before starting a new diet or eating plan.

WHO SHOULD FAST?

Some people are likely to see more results from intermittent fasting than others. This includes people who:

•Want something easy to follow

•ARE CONSTANTLY HUNGRY

If you are someone who frequently overeats or is always snacking throughout the day, intermittent fasting can help you promote healthier eating habits. If you're only allowed to eat at certain periods of time, you are telling your body not to release ghrelin (the hunger hormone) all the time. This balances your body's hormones, which curbs your appetite and causes you to feel less hungry throughout the day.

•AT RISK OF DEVELOPING DIABETES

If you are pre-diabetic and are at risk of developing diabetes, intermittent fasting may be beneficial. People who are prediabetic are likely to be insulin resistant. This means the body's cells are no longer sensitive to insulin. As a result, the body's blood sugar levels will continue to remain high following a meal. Fasting may help to reduce blood sugar levels and improve insulin resistance.

•WANT TO LOSE SOME EXTRA WEIGHT

Fasting has been shown to be an extremely effective weight loss tool. Research has shown that people who fast lose more weight and fat on average than people who don't fast. This is due to the reason that fasting helps to boost your metabolism and force your body to burn the fat reserves for fuel instead of sugar or muscle.

IS IT SAFE FOR WOMEN TO FAST?

Although fasting is safe, fasting may affect men and women differently. For instance, research shows that fasting helps to improve insulin sensitivity in men; however, can make blood sugar levels worse in women. There have been cases where women's menstrual cycles have stopped during their fasts. However, after they went back to regular eating, their menstrual cycles returned back to normal. Women who are pregnant, breastfeeding, trying to conceive, or have had fertility problems should avoid going on an intermittent fast.

One fasting method that may be worth trying is the Crescendo Method. The Crescendo Method is more gentle on your body and better for hormonal balance. The person would fast for 12-16 hours,

2-3 days a week instead of fasting every day for 12-20 hours. The fasting days should be non-consecutive, for example, Monday, Wednesday, and Friday. This fasting method has shown to be effective for many women and may show that women may not need to fast as long to get the same benefits as men.

On your fasting days, physical activities should be limited to light exercises, such as walking and yoga. Be sure to keep yourself hydrated and pay attention to your body. If you experience any abnormal changes to your period cycles, stop fasting immediately and consult with your doctor.

ARE YOU ALLOWED TO DRINK LIQUIDS WHILE FASTING?

Yes! Liquids such as water, coffee, tea are great and will help you to feel full between meals. Coffee and tea are appetite suppressants. You can add small amounts of milk or cream to your coffee or tea; however, sugar is not allowed.

Soda, pop, juice, and other calorie-ladened drinks are not allowed while fasting. These sweetened beverages are often packed with sugar and calories. These extra calories can add up, making it harder to lose those extra pounds.

I HEARD THAT SKIPPING BREAKFAST IS BAD. IS THIS TRUE?

No, this is not necessarily true. Previously, it was believed that breakfast helps to lower your food intake later in the day. However, research shows that skipping breakfast does not decrease the body's metabolism, nor does it cause people to eat more during lunch or dinner.

If you find yourself overeating later in the day, you should take a look at your diet. If you are eating lots of processed or high-sugary foods, you will get hungry sooner than if you were to eat foods high in protein and fiber.

Is it unsafe to fast for long periods of time?

Fasting is not only safe but is great for your overall health. It boosts your metabolism, promotes fat loss, and improves insulin sensitivity and blood sugar levels. The biggest issue for most people is that they're overeating as opposed to eating too little. We're constantly eating throughout the day. This overeating has led to an obesity epidemic in the states and most of the western world. Intermittent fasting isn't about denying your body calories and nutrients. Instead, it is about getting your calories and nutrients at a specific time period. Fasting gives your body a break from the constant insulin spike and sugar rush of food. This creates better eating habits and promotes weight loss for your body.

Are we allowed to fast and workout?

Yes, you can combine your intermittent fasting and workout routine. The act of fasting makes your body more resilient by putting stress on your body (in a good way). So, if you work out too intensely, you may overstrain your body. Hence, it's better to stick to light cardio exercises, such as walking and yoga on fasting days. You can do more intense workouts, like weight training or HIIT, on your non-fasting days.

On the other hand, there is some research that shows working out in a fasted-state can boost your metabolism and HGH production. If you are just starting out, I recommend starting off slowly before doing more intense workouts so you don't overstrain yourself. Always listen to your body. If you feel lightheaded or weak during your workout, stop and give yourself a break.

• • •

IS IT NECESSARY TO FAST EVERY DAY?

Of course not. The great thing about intermittent fasting is that it can be adapted to your schedule. Whether you can fast every day or only once or twice a week, fasting intermittently is still beneficial to your health. The key is to test, tweak, and stick with a fasting schedule that works for you.

AM I ALLOWED TO TAKE SUPPLEMENTS WHILE FASTING?

Yes, it's fine. Just be sure to follow the directions on the bottle as some supplements have to be taken with food.

IS FASTING SAFE FOR SENIORS?

Some studies indicate that fasting can help improve cognitive health and promote new brain cells to grow. This keeps the brain sharp and may help to protect against degenerative diseases (Alzheimer's, dementia and Huntington's) which becomes more prevailent as we get older. To be safe, always speak to your physician and health care provider to ensure fasting is a safe option for you.

DOES FASTING REALLY HELP YOU TO LIVE LONGER?

Although much research needs to be done, there is some indication that fasting may help to increase one's lifespan. One study examined how intermittent fasting affected rats' overall health. Rats were given different fasting schedules: fasting every other day, once every three days, or once every four days. Another group of rats was put on a regular feeding schedule.

The male rats who fasted every other day and female rats who fasted every three days showed the best health improvements. Interestingly enough, all the rats who were on a fasting schedule weighed less and lived longer than rats who were on a regular feeding schedule.

WON'T FASTING CAUSE MY BODY TO ENTER STARVATION MODE?

No, this will not happen since most intermittent fasting methods only ask you to fast for 24 hours or less. You would have to fast for weeks on end before your body begins to starve. Most people eat every few hours. By eating so frequently, the body is constantly burning carbs and sugars from the food rather than the body's fat. Fasting allows your body to burn fat instead of food. Thus, it's crazy to think that your body will enter starvation mode only after a few hours of fasting.

Many short-term diets focus on depriving your body of food to lose weight. Although this may work initially, your body will eventually enter starvation mode and have a harder time losing weight as the body clings to fat to keep functioning. During this time, your leptin levels will deplete (the appetite suppression hormone) and ghrelin levels will rise (the body's hunger hormones). This increases your risks of overeating on your next meal to satisfy your cravings.

By depriving your body of food periodically, fasting forces your body to use its stored fat as energy. In fact, in 1965, an extremely overweight male, weighing at 456 pounds was able to lose more than half his weight (275 pounds) after fasting for 382 days. That is over one year of fasting!

WHAT IS THE DIFFERENCE BETWEEN A FED STATE AND A FASTED state?

A fed state occurs during the period you are eating, digesting, and absorbing food. The fed state can last anywhere from 3-5 hours as your body is digesting the food. During this time, your body's insulin levels are elevated, which reduces your body's ability to burn fat.

12 hours after your meal, your body will enter a fasted state. During the fasted stated, your body's insulin levels will fall and your body is able to burn fat since its no longer using its resources to digest and absorb food. Fasting for longer periods, such as at least 16 hours, has been shown to increase your metabolism and make it easier to burn fat.

WHAT DOES THE TYPICAL INTERMITTENT FASTING DAY LOOK LIKE?

Although most people's days will vary, people who follow the 16:8 diet will usually skip breakfast and eat their first meal around noon. They will eat their meals between 12 pm and 8 pm after which they will fast until 12 pm the next day. Some people choose to eat a few bigger meals during the 8-hour eating window while others may eat many smaller meals.

ARE WE ALLOWED TO EAT AS MANY TIMES AS WE WANT DURING THE 8-hour feeding window?

Yes, you can eat as often as you want during your feeding window. It is up to you whether you want to eat two big meals for lunch and dinner or if you want to just snack throughout the day, either is fine.

However, you shouldn't go crazy and overeat. Eat until you are 90-95% full. Since you're limiting your meals within a shorter time frame, it makes it more difficult to overeat. So, unless you're dramatically increasing your calorie consumption, you're likely going to lose weight while still eating normally.

. . .

WHAT IF I GET HUNGRY?

Feeling hungry is one of the common challenges that people struggle with when fasting. Your hunger pains will be stronger during the first few days; however, they will gradually subside over time. In fact, most people notice that their appetite gets smaller after a few days of intermittent fasting.

The key to dealing with hunger is to stay busy. Oftentimes, we will eat or notice we are hungry when we are bored or not doing anything. Instead of focusing on the hunger, keep yourself busy. Take a walk, do some yoga, or meet up with a friend. Also, drinking water, coffee, or tea will help you feel full between meals.

WON'T I LOSE MUSCLE MASS IF I FAST?

You should be able to retain most of your muscle mass unless you are severely restricting your calories for long periods of time. Since most people will be breaking their fasts within a 24-hour period, you will be giving your body the essential nutrients it needs to refuel and retain muscle.

Research shows that fasting can actually improve energy and performance. This can help you get more from your workouts. Many athletes and bodybuilders incorporate fasting as part of their diet to optimize their physical performance. Other studies show that human growth hormone (HGH) levels increase when fasting, which helps to keep you strong. To preserve muscle mass, be sure to incorporate weight training and consume plenty of protein.

WHEN SHOULD I START TO SEE RESULTS?

This will highly depend on your body, health, diet, genetics, and lifestyle. However, most people should start seeing physical differences within the first few weeks. If you do not see any noticeable results after this time, do not be discouraged. Keep at it. Weight loss should not be a race to drop as many pounds as quickly as possible. Instead, it's something that should be planned out and happen gradually over time. Aim to lose 1-2 lbs a week.

WHAT IS THE SECRET TO LONG-TERM WEIGHT LOSS?

There is no secret. Losing weight takes hard work, patience, and commitment. If it was that easy, we would all be fitness models while eating Cheetos and donuts every day. Once you are able to figure out what your body needs, you will be more likely to reach your weight loss goals. Begin by changing your eating habits, getting more exercise, and making healthier lifestyle choices. If you want to lose weight (and keep it off), you can't be doing what you've always done and expect different results. In order to create change, you have to change your actions. And that all starts with making a commitment to living a better healthier life.

THREE

The Science of Intermittent Fasting

ou've learned a lot about Intermittent Fasting so far, but you still likely don't understand why it all works so well for dieting and health. This chapter is the antidote to that confusion! You will learn how Intermittent Fasting affect the body, how it interacts with diabetes, heart health, aging, and finally, the female body. By the end of this chapter, you should feel both highly informed about IF and aware of a few potential complications.

How IF Affects the Body

When you're feeling hungry, your body is under the sway of two very important hormones: leptin and ghrelin, and Intermittent Fasting affects both of those hormones substantially. In a typical situation, leptin decreases sensations of being hungry, and ghrelin makes you feel hungry instead. While leptin is secreted from fat cells throughout the body, ghrelin is only secreted from the stomach's lining. Together, leptin and ghrelin communicate with the brain's hypothalamus, telling the body when to stop or start eating. During IF, these hormones are released less often, causing the body to have a whole different experience of hunger and fullness.

Another important hormone in the context of eating and hunger suppression is insulin itself. The pancreas produces insulin, and it regulates how much glucose exists in our blood. Ultimately, high or low amounts of insulin affect the individual's weight greatly. Too little insulin and one can't keep weight on. Too much insulin and one can't lose weight whatsoever. While it seems that lower insulin is desired, there has to be a healthy balance, for too low insulin is actually disastrous for the body since glucose (or blood sugar) is a large part of how the body gets energy.

ONE FINAL INFLUENCER OF THE BODY'S HUNGER AND WEIGHT LOSS situation is the individual's thyroid. If the thyroid is overactive, metabolism will work quickly, and energy, health, and weight will be affected. Conversely, an underactive thyroid will slow metabolism, energy, and health, and it will contribute to increased weight.

IN THE END, INTERMITTENT FASTING AFFECTS THE INDIVIDUAL'S weight by varying the production of these three important hormones and by working with the thyroid's natural potential. Essentially, those practicing IF will trigger these hormones to be released less often (or more consistently if the person is obese or diabetic to start with) due to the less-frequent eating schedule. Eventually, even the thyroid's effects should become balanced out through this altered eating schedule.

IF and Diabetes

For people with diabetes, Intermittent Fasting poses certain risks as well as incredible benefits. People with diabetes have altered insulin levels compared to the non-diabetic person, due to insulin resistance in their bodies. People with Type 1 diabetes cannot make insulin. They need to take insulin daily to have the energy and vigor to live. People with Type 2 diabetes have bodies that don't produce much insulin or don't use that insulin well at all.

With these altered productions of insulin, the blood sugar levels of the body have no way to be regulated, meaning that there's more standing glucose in the blood at all times with no way for it to get into the cells to be used for natural and physical energy. This higher blood sugar level can cause additional problems for the individual over time, but there is no legitimate cure other than taking insulin daily.

Intermittent Fasting, however, can provide a temporary cure when applied correctly in the lives of diabetic individuals (whose diabetic conditions are not severe). When IF is done on a daily basis with just a few fasting hours a day, people with diabetes show improved weight, blood sugar levels, and standing glucose levels. These individuals are not recommended to skip entire meals or fast for days at a time. Also, is not recommended for these people to strictly diet while they're applying IF. Instead, it works better to make food portions smaller and to eat fewer snacks in between.

IF and Heart Health

Heart health is a complicated issue in today's world. We all want to be healthy and thrive, but the foods we eat and the activities we engage in often don't align with those goals, and those more immediate actions win out. In effect, many of our hearts aren't as healthy as they could be. Heart disease is still the biggest killer in the world to this day. However, the introduction of Intermittent Fasting into someone's lifestyle can greatly alter this potential, for it can reduce many risks associated with heart disease.

. . .

FOR EXAMPLE, RECENT STUDIES DONE ON ANIMALS HAVE PROVED that the practice of Intermittent Fasting improves numerous risk factors for heart disease. Some of these improvements include lowered cholesterol, reduced inflammation in the body, balanced blood sugar levels, and lower blood pressure. Essentially, IF won't cure heart disease, but it will reduce several risk factors that may exist in one's body (with or without him or her knowing).

WHEN IT COMES DOWN TO IT, AS LONG AS ONE'S INTERMITTENT Fasting experience involves the reintroduction of electrolytes into the body, there's no potential harm posed to the heart whatsoever. There's only potential for growth, bolstering, and strengthening. However, without the right reintroduction of electrolytes, there is still the possibility of heart palpitations in individuals attempting IF. The heart needs electrolytes for its stability and efficacy, so as long as you drink a bit of salt with your water, your heart will only thank you!

IF and Aging

People love to talk about how Intermittent Fasting can reverse the effects of aging, and they're not wrong! The tricky part is elucidating the science behind the process they're referencing. The anti-aging potential tied up with Intermittent Fasting applies mostly to two things: 1) your brain and 2) your whole body, through what's called "autophagy."

OVERALL, INTERMITTENT FASTING HEALS THE BODY THROUGH ITS ability to rejuvenate the cells. With this restricted caloric intake due to eating schedule or timing, the body's cells can function with less limitation and confusion while producing more energy for the body to use. In effect, the cells function more efficiently while the body can burn more fat and take in more oxygen for the organs and blood, encouraging the individual to live longer with increased sensations of "youth."

About those two original examples, Intermittent Fasting has been proven 1) to keep the brain fit and agile. It improves overall cognitive function and memory capacity as well as cleverness, wit, and quick, clear thinking in the moment. Furthermore, Intermittent Fasting 2) keeps the cells fit and agile through autophagy (which is kickstarted by IF), where the cells are encouraged to clean themselves up and get rid of any "trash" that might be clogging up the works. By just restricting your eating schedule a little bit each day (or each week), you can find your brain power boosted and your body ready for anything.

IF and the Female Body

Intermittent Fasting requires a different technique than most diets do, which is why it's more often referred to as a lifestyle. Additionally, this variance means that the effects of IF on the female body are a little different than the effects of the standard diet. For instance, dieting will easily cause weight loss in most people, but IF is a little trickier and much less consistent for women especially.

The female body, being created with birthing potential, has specific needs that are altered through an Intermittent Fasting eating schedule. With less hormones being released (which tell women when they are hungry and full) there is less fat being stored in their bodies and less fertility when it comes to their later aims of reproducing. In combination with a strict diet that counts calories or restricts fats, Intermittent Fasting can be dangerous for women of all ages.

For women who still want to work with Intermittent Fasting, there's a lot of hope left for you! Just make sure to follow these four steps to ensure that you're doing it in the most healthy way for your body and your future children. First, make sure you're very connected to your body. You'll want to be very aware if something on the inside seems "off" or "wrong" (bodily, emotionally, and mentally), especially considering all that's at stake, hormonally and reproductively.

Second, make serious effort to be aware of your body's cycles and note when things go askew. Without the right awareness of your menstruation, you risk going a long time with an altered cycle. This alteration might not sound like a lot, but it can affect many different aspects of your body and your childrearing potential.

Third, please don't try to combine strict dieting and Intermittent Fasting. I know you want to be fit and strong and slim, but you still want to make sure you're getting enough fat and calories, considering what your body is able to do with these right amounts of fat and calories.

Fourth and finally, make sure you're also not exercising too ferociously while you first transition to Intermittent Fasting. If you've been trying IF as a lifestyle for a while, you're welcome to add fitness and exercise back into the mix, but it is really dangerous for the female body to combine two intense practices at once. I understand the urge to lose weight and be healthy, but you'll need to make sure you're not eliminating too much from your body at any given time.

FOUR

Intermittent Fasting and Exercise

W hen it comes to intermittent fasting, it is important to understand how it will affect your ability to exercise if you plan on sticking with the practice in the long-term. The biggest difference you will notice when you are exercising while fasting is that you will naturally feel weaker as less food in your stomach means less available fuel for building new muscles during an exercise routine. As such, if you do plan on exercising regularly while practicing any form of intermittent fasting it is important to take a number of extra precautions in order to ensure your new dietary habits don't end up negatively impacting the effectiveness of your average workout.

TEN MUSCLE BIOPSIES WERE TAKEN BEFORE EXERCISE, AS WELL AS three hours after exercise. The results showed that exercising while in a glycogen depleted state was able to increase mitochondrial biogenesis. This is the process by which new mitochondria can form inside the cells. The authors of the study believe that exercising on a low glycogen level diet may be beneficial for improving muscle oxidative capacity.

EXERCISE AND INTERMITTENT FASTING BASICS

Regardless if you are looking to improve your strength or your endurance, it is important to keep in mind that fats don't burn as easily as carbs do which means you are going to have less access to immediate energy. On the plus side, however, you will find that you are able to last much longer overall. This is also why you are likely to burn about 20 percent more fat when exercising without carbs in your system than you otherwise would. This is also why you should exercise immediately prior to breaking your fast as opposed to once it has been broken.

UNFORTUNATELY, THE BODY DOESN'T JUST LOOK FOR EXTRA FAT when it needs energy while exercising, it also requires available protein as well. As protein is stored in your muscles, if you exercise too strenuously then you will actually be hurting your muscles as opposed to helping them. You should be able to get through a moderate exercise routine without risk, however, as long as you don't push it too far. Thus, you should leave the heavier workouts for days when you are consuming more calories on a regular basis.

THIS MEANS THAT ONCE YOUR BODY ADAPTS TO ITS NEW ROUTINE you will naturally have more energy left over for things like exercise in addition to all of your core bodily functions. You can expect it to take about a month for your body to fully adapt to the process. When it comes to merging your existing exercise plan with intermittent fasting, it is vital that you keep in mind that all types of exercise are going to be more difficult right off the bat than what you may remember while your body adjusts to the transition.

This is perfectly natural, of course, you are exercising on an empty stomach after all. Due to the fact that your blood sugar levels and glycogen levels are going to be lower than normal as well, you will likely feel weaker to start to boot. This means it is extremely important to schedule your workout at the appropriate time depending on the goals you have set for yourself. Just make sure you are giving your body the tools it needs to take advantage of all of your hard work.

Exercise tips

What to eat: Sometimes, you will wake up feeling weak instead of ready to start exercising. On these days, you should eat something small before getting started, such as a handful of nuts or a piece of fruit. It's advisable to have a small meal with simple carbs and some protein, such as a protein shake with a banana, or a simple protein bar. If you aren't able to have that much, even a glass of juice can help you make it through your exercise plan more easily in the morning.

If you only have about 30 minutes before your workout, try to pick solid foods that will digest as quickly as possible and limit fiber since it can be rough on your digestive process. If you do decide to work out in a fasted state, always bring some easily digested food just in case. As always, water is extremely important, so make sure you get plenty of that both before, during, and after any physical activity.

. . .

PRIORITIZE LOW-INTENSITY CARDIO: IF YOU PLAN ON EXERCISING regularly while you are fasting, it is important to limit your cardio to low-intensity options. This means you should still be able to carry on a conversation with relative ease if you are exercising during a fast. Ideally, you are going to want to stick to things like a light jog or 25 minutes on a cardio machine and be sure not to push yourself too hard. It will also be extra important to listen to your body and take a breather if you start to feel dizzy or light-headed which is going to happen much more often than it otherwise would. If you ignore this advice and push your exercise intensity level to the limit then it will make the rest of your workout feel like much more of a struggle regardless of what you are doing.

CHOOSE YOUR BATTLES: THIS IS NOT TO SAY THAT YOU SHOULD never push your body to the limit while fasting. Instead, it is important to time your more intense periods of exercise to about an hour after you have eaten. This will give your body time to process the nutrients you have provided for it and will help you to maximize the amount of fat you can lose while still staying properly fueled for the workout by having plenty of glycogen in your system which will also help to reduce the risk of low blood sugar levels. Additionally, if you can afford to alter your fasting schedule slightly, following up a high-intensity workout with a snack that is high in carbs is also encouraged because your muscles will have burned through the available glycogen while still being hungry for more.

UP YOUR PROTEIN INTAKE: STANDARD WORKOUT CONVENTION suggest that you are going to want to take in between 20 and 30 grams of protein every four hours while you are awake. While intermittent fasting makes this unattainable, you're should still aim to take in between 80 and 120 grams of protein per day. If you are planning a serious strength workout then you should plan to do so between two snacks, if not two full meals.

EXERCISES TO START WITH WHILE FASTING

What follows are a few exercises of the sort you should aim for when exercising while fasting, at least to start. As previously noted, you can certainly take the time to push yourself but starting with exercises like these will get your body used to exercising while fasting without putting you at risk in the process.

DYNAMIC STRETCHING: AFTER YOU HAVE THE BLOOD PUMPING BUT before you start the workout proper it is important to stretch well to prevent injury.

•Head Circles: Start with your chin facing downwards and rotate your head in a gentle circle in both a clockwise and counter-clockwise direction.

•Shoulder Circles: Start with your hand at your sides and slowly roll your shoulders first in one direction and then the other. Ensure your chest and upper back work together.

•Arm Circles: Stretch your arms out and start by making small circles with your arms, gradually expanding until the circumference of the circles extends to include your ears and your hips.

•Torso Circles: Stretch your arms out to the sides and twist your core in one direction and then the other as far as you can without straining yourself.

•Leg Circles: Start by lying on your back with your forearms pressed against the floor. Place one leg straight out and the other bent at the knee while making circles in the air.

Butterflies: For this exercise, you can stand. Bring your hands by your ears so that the elbows are bent, and bend over so that your back is flat. Next, lift the elbows away from the ears, making sure that the shoulder blades are pushing towards one another. Repeat this exercise for at least thirty reps, because of the fact that you will not be using weights. If you want to experience more intensity, using weights for this exercise will certainly intensify the workout.

Kick-ups: To begin this exercise you will want to get on your hands and knees so that your weight is supported by both your knees and your forearms. You will then alternate between legs as you lift one leg off of the ground and kick backwards so your heels face upwards. You will then return the leg to the starting position in one fluid motion. This exercise is beneficial to both the core and the legs.

Hip Bridge: To begin this exercise you will want to lay on your back so that your knees are bent and both of your feet are planted firmly on the floor. You will then want to lift your hips as far off the ground as possible, while at the same time clenching your buttocks, with the end goal being to create a perfectly straight line between your knees as your shoulders. If you are interested in making this exercise even more difficult you can instead aim to keep one foot on the floor while at the same time lifting the other so that it points at the ceiling. This exercise is great for improving hip flexibility while at the same time stretching the spine and improving back strength.

PLANK: TO BEGIN THIS EXERCISE YOU WILL WANT TO GET ON YOUR hands and knees before placing all of your weight on your forearms and balancing on your toes. After you are in the position you will then want to tense your entire body, placing special focus on your core, and hold that position for as long as possible. While this might seem simple on the surface, once you try it you will be surprised at just how strenuous it can be. This exercise is useful in strengthening the core.

SUPERMAN: TO PERFORM THIS EXERCISE YOU WILL WANT TO LAY FACE down on the ground with your arms out in front of you and your legs straight. You will then simply lift both your arms and legs off the ground at the same time, as high as you can. During this exercise you will want to keep your arms and legs stable rather than moving up and down, you will also want to hold for as long as possible. This is a great exercise when it comes to strengthening your back.

ELLIPTICAL TRAINER: USING AN ELLIPTICAL TRAINER FOR 45 MINUTES will burn roughly 330 calories or just shy of three-fourths of what you need to burn in a day to lose 1-2 pounds a week when eating about 1,500 calories per day. This piece of exercise equipment is extremely low impact while still being fairly good at burning calories. If you can find a version that offers an arm as well as leg component, you can burn even more calories at once.

. . .

Go for a swim: Swimming at a decent clip for as little as 45 minutes will burn roughly 340 calories or almost 75 percent of what you need to burn in a day to lose 1-2 pounds a week when eating about 1,500 calories per day. Swimming is a great choice for exercising if you have joint issues, are overweight or suffer from arthritis as the water helps minimize pain related to resistance. Start at a slow pace for thirty minutes at a go and work up from there.

Ride a bike: Riding a bike at a decent pace for as little as 45 minutes will burn roughly 380 calories or almost 80 percent of what you need to burn in a day to lose 1-2 pounds a week when eating about 1,500 calories per day. This classic exercise lets you get some fresh air while stretching your muscles and is a great way to ease yourself into an exercise routine. If you plan on riding a bike for exercise it is important to purchase one that is properly fitted to reduce soreness and the chance of injury.

FIVE

Getting Started with Intermittent Fasting

B efore beginning intermittent fasting, you might want to consider consulting your doctor or dietitian first. Make an appointment to see your doctor for a check-up and get some blood work done at the time.

PREPARE YOURSELF MENTALLY AND PHYSICALLY BEFORE GETTING started. When you first begin fasting, your body might react and be a little shocked at first. You may see some side effects. We will discuss this in more detail shortly. Plan to track your results. Monitor your body for changes and continue to track your blood work.

AFTER THAT, GETTING STARTED WITH INTERMITTENT FASTING IS A very easy process! The easiest way to start is to do a bit of research, choose a method that works well with your lifestyle, and give it a try! As you ease into fasting, experiment with the different approaches. Find a schedule that works for you and fits your lifestyle. Keep in mind that you don't really need to follow a structured plan as you get started. An alternative is to fast whenever you would like to. Try skipping meals from time to time when you don't feel hungry or don't have a lot of time to prepare or eat a meal.

INTERMITTENT FASTING IS AN EASY LIFESTYLE TO ADOPT. BELOW, WE will look at a few tips and recommendations that will increase your knowledge and your chances of being successful.

TIPS FOR SUCCESS

•SOME STUDIES INDICATE THAT INTERMITTENT FASTING MAY NOT BE quite as beneficial for women as it is for men. Fasting may affect men and women differently. Women may be more sensitive to calorie restriction, and some may have less significant results in regard to weight loss. Fasting may also affect hormone production that is needed for the reproductive cycle. Some women report that their menstrual period stopped when they started doing intermittent fasting. Women may need to make some adjustments and consider a modified approach to fasting. It might best to start with shorter fasting periods and to do them less often. Experiment and see what works best. Listen to your body and stop immediately if you experience the absence of menstruation.

•Stay busy—try not to hyper-focus on when you will eat next or how hungry you are. This will make the fasting periods more difficult. Plan to spend a large chunk of your fasting hours asleep or preoccupied with other thoughts and things.

•Have a well-balanced approach to all other aspects of your life. This should include spending time doing things that you enjoy and participating in exercise and social engagements. Intermittent fasting should work well with your life. It should not add confusion or complications.

•Manage hunger by riding out the hunger pains. Recognize that the hunger will pass. Hunger tends not to build and build until you eat. It is more likely to come in waves. Do not worry or think too much about it when you do feel hungry.

•Understand that your body will not go into starvation mode by fasting for a day or two at a time. It is a common misunderstanding that when we do not eat for prolonged periods, our body will start to store calories rather than burn them. There is no scientific evidence for this. In actuality, it takes many days and a dramatic amount of starvation before our body kicks into starvation mode. The fasting schedules that we are discussing in this book do not apply to circumstances such as this.

•Drink plenty of water. Water is good for you and may help ease some of your hunger pains as you get used to the new eating schedule.

•Track your progress. Keep notes on your weight and your performance. If you are concerned about weight loss, try tracking your calories for a week or two to see if you are taking in too many during non-fasting periods.

•Drink coffee or tea, but only in moderation—and do not add sugar. It is a good idea to be cautious of caffeinated drinks in general and try not to rely on them as a meal replacement. Consuming too much caffeine while fasting can disrupt your circadian rhythm during fasting periods. Other zero-calorie beverages are okay too like diet soda or sparkling water.

•Eat a well-balanced diet when you are not fasting. If you are hoping to increase the rate at which you are losing weight, combine your fasting with a low-carb diet. Focus on eating lots of fruit and vegetables and high-quality protein. Cut back on junk food and processed food for better results.

•Also, don't binge after fasting. It is a much better idea to break your fast gently. The longer the fast, the more careful you should be easing in. Eating an oversized meal after any length of fast can cause an upset stomach.

•Relax and try not to overthink things. Your fasting schedule does not need to be perfect of followed to a tee. It does not need to be as cut and dry as this. Remember to be flexible and do what works for you. Don't overthink things and keep things simple. By having this frame of mind, you will be more likely to stick with intermittent fasting and see better results.

•Exercise. It is perfectly okay to keep up your normal exercise routine while fasting. If you are new to exercise, try starting with brisk walks each day and work your way up to more strenuous activities. Be sure to listen to your body during workouts of any type. If you get lightheaded, stop. Drink plenty of fluids to ease into fasted workouts.

•Try to stick with it! Give yourself a month of fasting before expecting too many results or trying something else.

POTENTIAL SIDE EFFECTS

WITH ANY TYPE OF CHANGE IN DIET, HABITS, OR LIFESTYLE, YOU MAY experience physical or mental side effects. It is important to be aware of the possible side effects before you start your fast. In general, there seem to be very few negative side effects for those who implement an intermittent fasting program.

· · ·

HUNGER PAINS ARE THE MOST COMMON SIDE EFFECT OF intermittent fasting. Food cravings may go along with this, as well as being over-focused on your non-fasting windows. Some people deal with mood swings while fasting and dizziness or reduced energy levels at the beginning.

YOU MAY EXPERIENCE DIFFICULTY CONCENTRATING OR SOME "BRAIN fog." These symptoms are usually mild and tend to go away after a few cycles of fasting. Diarrhea or constipation may be a side effect for some people, and headaches are fairly common. Symptoms such as these are usually just temporary and will slowly disappear once your body has had time to adapt to the new meal schedule.

HEARTBURN MAY OCCUR AS YOUR BODY GETS USED TO INTERMITTENT fasting. Some people have also reported other side effects such as bad breath on fasting days or feeling overly full following first meal after a fast.

WHO SHOULD NOT FAST

•WOMEN WHO ARE PREGNANT, BREASTFEEDING, OR TRYING TO conceive should not fast as these are not the times to attempt weight loss.

•Anyone with a history of eating disorders like anorexia or bulimia should also avoid fasting. The restricted diet may become a trigger for relapse.

•Those who are underweight, malnourished, or have nutritional deficiencies also should not attempt this approach.

•Fasting is not recommended for children under the age of 18. Children and teenagers still need extra nutrients to grow.

•If you have a diagnosed medical condition, it is best to consult with your doctor before trying intermittent fasting. Especially if you:

oHave diabetes or regularly experience low blood sugar levels. Intermittent fasting is generally not recommended for those who have been prescribed blood sugar–lowering medications.

oAre a woman with fertility problems or a history of missed periods.

oHave a condition called Familial Hypercholesterolemia.

oHave low blood pressure.

oHave gout or high uric acid.

oTake medications. You first need to make sure that fasting will not have a negative impact on any medication you might be taking or negatively impact any health concerns—for example, medication that you are required to take every morning with food.

ALL THAT BEING SAID, INTERMITTENT FASTING IS A VERY SAFE method of losing weight and improving health. There is nothing dangerous about not eating for a while if you are otherwise healthy and in good physical condition.

Afterword

As we have seen, intermittent fasting has a wide range of health benefits. As more research is carried out and we learn more about this form of eating, we can learn how to use it to improve our quality of life.

In the end, consistency is the only thing that will help you reach your goals. Although making changes to your diet and lifestyle may take hard work and persistence, I believe it's worth it. Health is the more precious thing in life. Once you lose it, it's extremely difficult to get it back. By taking the necessary steps to protect your health, you will be able to live life to the fullest.

Thank you again for reading this book and I wish you all the best in your weight loss journey. Happy fasting!

www.ingramcontent.com/pod-product-compliance
Lightning Source LLC
Chambersburg PA
CBHW051132250726
48655CB00007B/3009